KETO FOR WOMEN OVER 50

Your Essential Guide to Lose Weight, Feel Younger and Live a Healthy Lifestyle After 50.

By Jason Smith

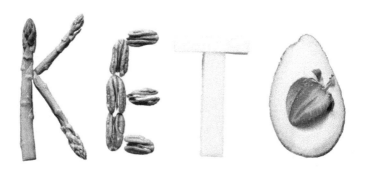

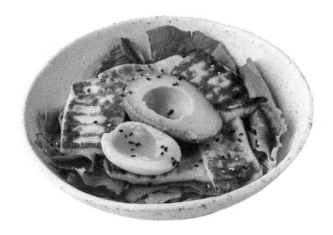

Table of contents

12) Bacon & Halloumi Sausages 54

13) Pork in Garlic & Red Wine 55

14) Pan-Seared Pork & Pepper 56

15) Zucchini & Sausage Stew 56

16) Mediterranean Meatballs & Mozzarella 58

17) Salmon & Pistachio Hot Pot 59

18) Chicken with Onion Mayo 60

19) Beef & Tomato Pie 61

20) Aromatic Spinach & Cheese Curry 62

21) Keto baked apples 63

22) Keto bagel recipe 64

23) Keto southwestern breakfast skillet 64

24) Keto Banana Pancakes 66

25) Keto BLT lettuce wraps 67

26) Cream cheese scrambled eggs 67

27) Keto coconut porridge 68

28) Keto Sausage with Creamy Basil Sauce 69

29) Cheesy Keto garlic bread 70

30) Keto seeded bread 72

31) Paleo and keto butter chicken 73

32) Baked Artichoke Hearts Au Gratin 75

33) Chicken green curry 76

34) Keto beef kabobs 78

35) Super simple braised red cabbage 79

36) Labneh cheese ball 80

37) Keto Caesar salad 81

38) Chicken, spinach, and bacon salad 83

39) Keto broccoli salad 84

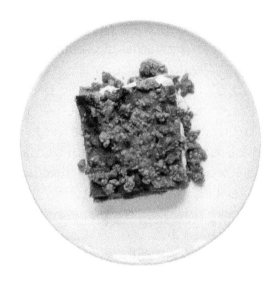

Introduction

Amongst living in what is considered a 'technologically advanced' 21st century, the hectic nature of day to day life often causes man to disregard the important factors that allow us to function the way we do; specifically our internal health. According to recent statistics, it is acknowledged that over 50% of employment is digitalized therefore justifying the ideology that obesity is a grave issue due to the lack of physical movement and interaction man has. Although a workout method may be suggested, it is of no use unless supported alongside a corresponding diet which would ensure that any fat is burnt properly and efficiently- This is something websites won't tell you.

Nowadays, it is fairly common to see the craze of salads doing wonders for the body; flat stomachs, idealistic bodies, sound perfect right? Although it has its benefits, such as providing nutrients to the body to stimulate powerful antioxidants in the blood- it does very little to reduce body mass. After years of research to find a diet plan that not only brings about good eating habits but also solves this issue equally as well, man has bought about a concept known as the "keto diet."In reality, theconcept was based around issues such as cancers, epilepsy, and Alzheimer's, and it was believed that keto wondered enabled the prevention of cells from gaining their energy from glucose (blood sugar); however, over time, many who had used this prog took notice of the weight loss advantages during participation, therefore,labeling this diet as what we now know to be a 'weight loss prog.'

Alongside the benefit of eating well, this diet is believed to encourage a regular and orderly eating schedule, which proves to be challenging in this day and age. However, normally our bodies would use our carbohydrate stores to provide the service of breaking down fats and play a role as a provider of energy. Still, in this case, the lack of carbohydrate intake due to this diet would force our bodies to extract energy from fat stores, which is a system known as 'Ketosis.'

Keto is most suited to those over 50 specifically because that is a period where women undergo menopause in which women experience symptoms such as hormonal changes and a loss of appetite, and weight loss. Keto is believed to relieve mostmenopause symptoms due to its high fat and very low carb diet. However, during that period, it is also common to see a fluctuation in insulin levels. Keto is believed to help its sensitivity ensure a more controlled blood sugar level.

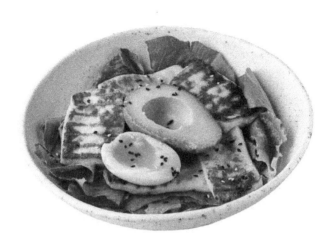

It helps the body more effectively burn its fat reserves. The ketogenic diet or keto diet involves removing carbohydrates from your diet and increasing fats. An eating plan that focuses on foods with lots of healthy fats, sufficient quantities of protein, and very few carbohydrates is a keto diet. The purpose is to promote more calories from fat than from carbohydrates. By depleting the body of its sugar stores, the diet operates. It will start to break down fat molecules for energy as a result. It contributes to the formation of molecules called ketones that the body uses for fuel. It may also cause weight loss as the body burns fat. The current study has shown that ketogenic diets are good for general health and weight loss.

1.1 How Ketogenic Diet Works?

Imagine your body as a car to understand why you could burn fat faster on a keto diet or be in ketosis. Your body breaks down food for energy into glucose: glucose is the petrol of your body.

What happens when the body doesn't have enough glucose to use? Your car does not run without fuel in any situation. Fortunately, it doesn't happen in your body as well. You have the replacement fuel known as ketones, created by your liver from fat that brings your body into a ketosis state. You reduce carbohydrates and protein on a keto diet;it suggests eating a diet high in fat. Insufficient protein or carbohydrates means you don't have a ton of glucose for food.The backup fuel is used by your body, turning the fat you consume and body fat into ketones.

You burn fat for food, literally

You still manufacture ketones. But if you consume a ketogenic diet, glucose is replaced by ketones as the dominant fuel for your body, and you get into ketosis. It moves from glucose to ketones for days or weeks, and controlling it is also equally difficult. Also, tiny quantities of carbohydrates or extra protein will prevent ketosis from being preserved by your body.

1.2 What is Ketosis?

Ketosis is a metabolic condition in which the body uses fat and ketones rather than glucose as the main energy source (sugar). In your liver, as required for nutrition, glucose is stored and released. After all, after carb intake has been exceptionally low for one to 2 days, this glucose supply becomes depleted. The brain needs an adequate supply of fuel to function continuously, but the mechanism of 'gluconeogenesis' is not enough. That is where the liver produces glucose from the amino acids found within the ingested proteins.

1. The Ketosis process provides the body, specifically the brain, with an alternate source of energy. The body rapidly forms ketones during ketosis. Ketones, also known as ketone bodies, are formed exclusively from fat already present in your liver, eaten, and fat from your own body.

Beta-hydroxybutyrate (BHB), acetoacetate, and acetone are the primary forms of ketone species.

2. Ketones are formed daily in the liver when consuming a higher-carb diet. It normally occurs often overnight while sleeping but in small numbers. During this, glucose and insulin levels are forced to decrease; however, the liver is on a carb-restricted diet, pushing to increase its ketone output to supply energy to the brain efficiently.

3. Until your blood crosses a certain ketone level, you are assumed to have nutritional ketosis. The 'edge' of nutritional ketosis is known to have a minimum of 0.5 mmol/L of BHBB.

4. While both fasting and a keto diet are useful, it will become obvious that a keto diet is sustainable over long periods. Besides, individuals should adopt easily finally.

1.3. Ketosis vs. ketoacidosis

Ketosis and ketoacidosis are both have a different concept, but they sound identical. The word 'ketoacidosis,' a form of 1 DM complication, refers to diabetic ketoacidosis (DKA). It is an extremely life-threatening disease that leads to a dangerously high level of ketones and blood glucose. For ketosis and ketoacidosis, as well as ketone, development takes place. It is known that ketosis is typically stable, while ketoacidosis can be life-threatening.

This blend makes the blood extremely acidic, directly targetingsensory organs' functioning in the body, such as the liver and kidneys. If this is the case, it is of the highest concern that it is handled. It can occur very quickly with DKA. In just 24 hours, it has the potential to expand. For those with type 1 diabetes whose bodies lack insulin, it is most prevalent. Many things could be caused by DKA, which is similar to illness, poor nutrition, or not taking a proper insulin dose. Many with type 2 diabetes with little or no development of insulin in their body are at risk of developing DKA.

Ketosis is a metabolic mechanism that starts when the body is on a low carbohydrate diet. After this, ketone bodies are formed by the liver. In ketosis, the ketone body's level rises to 8 mmol/l without causing changes to the pH value. The ketone bodies' level is forced to rise to 20 mmol/l during ketoacidosis, resulting in reduced PH levels. Both ketoacidosis and ketosis, therefore, contain ketones but have distinct efficiencies.

1.4. What are ketone bodies?

When there is an insulin deficiency in the blood, different chemicals are produced by the body. Instead of using glucose, internal fat is also allowed to break down as an energy supplier (sugar). All ketone species considered toxic acid chemicals are acetone, acetoacetate, and beta-hydroxybutyrate. They move through the blood and into the urine. Another way in which the body can get rid of acetone in the lungs (respiration). Ketosis is when ketone bodies are found in the blood, and urine containing ketone bodies is ketonuria.

The production house for liver ketones will manufacture ketone molecules at about 185 gs per day. Acetoacetate is a subform of liver-assembled ketones, whereas beta-hydroxybutyrate is the predominant blood circulating ketone molecules. After their formation, these are combined with acetyl coenzyme A (CoA) and join the 'Krebs cycle.' The Krebs cycle is considered a part of the metabolic pathway that uses oxygen to burn fuel to generate energy in organisms' breathing.

It is where they are used to produce energy molecules.

1.5. Types of Ketogenic Diets

The Keto Diet allows low carbohydrates and high fats to be consumed. Consumers are prohibited from buying candy, processed foods, grain and vegetable products. If one succeeds in implementing the exact delineated diet plan, all those health benefits enjoyed by those who have adopted the keto diet before can certainly be enjoyed.

1. The Ketogenic Regular Diet, or SKD

Proteins, fats, and carbohydrates are primarily the foundation of a ketogenic diet. Although the concentration of carbohydrates is between 5 and 10 percent, the protein concentration in keto diets fluctuates between 15 and 20 percent. That of fat in keto diets is up to 75 percent. However, it would help if you concentrated on incorporating fat-rich meals and snacks into the diet plan while preparing your meals to frame a keto diet since, under a keto diet, you need to eat 150 gs of fat per day. Besides, the concentration of carbohydrates in diet foods must be kept as low as possible such that the daily intake limit of carbohydrates, which is 50 gs, cannot be exceeded.

2. The Ketogenic Targeted Diet, or TKDD

The Intended Ketogenic Diet micronutrient ratio comprises 10-15 percent of carbohydrates, 60-70 percent of fat, and 20 percent of protein. Athletes who often need to eat carbohydrates before or during a workout typically follow this diet. Unlike the regular keto diet strategy, high carbohydrates can be eaten in conjunction with the Planned Ketogenic Diet.

3. The Ketogenic Cyclic Diet, or CKD

Targeted Ketogenic diet macronutrient ratio is 5-10 percent of carbohydrates, 75 percent of fat, and 15-20 percent of protein when on keto days; otherwise, 50 percent of carbohydrates, 25 percent of protein, and 25 percent of fat are composed of the macronutrient throughout off 'days.' The main goal of the Targeted Ketogenic Diet is to provide relief for keto dieters to turn on and off from ketosis while enjoying the diet simultaneously

4. The TKD or High-Protein Ketogenic Diet

The High-Protein Ketogenic Diet's macronutrient ratio is 5-10 percent carbohydrates, 60-65 percent fat, and 30 percent protein. It is recommended that those who aspire to opt for this kind of diet eat 120 gs of protein in tandem with 130 gs of fat daily. Most people are drawn towards this type of Keto diet due to a higher concentration of proteins and limited fats than other Keto diets.

Keto is a diet for weight loss. Low-carb keto diets, however, offer women in their 50s some significant additional benefits. Those advantages include:

1. Reduced body fat

A lot of diets claim weight loss, but the weight is just water in many cases. Keto improves the burning of fat and has better outcomes than most of the other diets. Keto also targets abdominal fat preferentially, appropriately called visceral fat,

In women who are over 50, abdominal fat begins to increase. It increases the risk of stroke, cardiac arrest, and heart failure. Abdominal fat deposition is mainly due to the hormonal changes associated with menopause.

2. Increased sensitivity to insulin

Carbs are digested and converted into glucose. When eating carbohydrates, your body releases the hormone insulin to ferry glucose into your liver and muscles. However, with age, the body's sensitivity to insulin decreases, meaning that the glucose is more likely to be converted into and processed as fat, contributing to weight gain.

Low carb diets increase insulin sensitivity. It ensures that the few carbs that you eat will not turn into fat. Increased insulin sensitivity also helps to regulate the levels of blood glucose. Low blood glucose levels are inextricably related to better overall health and a decreased risk of type 2 diabetes.

3. Extent brain function

Menopausal women also encounter things like memory loss, mood swings, and difficulty focusing. It can also make them suffer from depression and anxiety. It's because estrogen levels, the primary female sex hormone, decrease during menopause, affecting the amount of glucose that enters your brain.

The keto diet gives your brain an additional source of fuel; ketones. On ketones and a low-carb diet, the brain functions better. Far less popular are problems like mood swings and memory loss.

A decreased risk of many neurological disorders is also associated with the keto diet, including Alzheimer's disease and Parkinson's disease, all of which are more common in people over 50 years of age.

4. Inflammation reduced

The process of aging could be difficult on your body. Menopausal women experienced knee and hip pain and headaches, and other non-specific forms of pain in the 1950s.

Keto is a greater diet, and certain fats are very helpful for calming inflammation. Healthy anti-inflammatory fats that can form part of the keto diet include the following:

- Olive Oil
- For example, oily fish, sardines, tuna, and salmon
- Avocados and Avocado Oil
- Walnuts

By comparison, foods such as refined carbohydrates, sugar, and processed foods are all associated with increased inflammation. These foods do not constitute part of the keto.

5. Improved lipid profile in blood

When approaching their 50s, many women experience elevated triglyceride levels. It could be the epitome of heart attacks.

However, Low carb diets have been proven to reduce triglycerides and LDL cholesterol while being high in fat, alongside increasing 'Healthy HDL cholesterol. These improvements are associated with better cardiovascular health and a decreased risk of heart disease.

6. Decreased Blood Pressure

Research shows that the blood pressure of women appears to be lower than that of men. However, as you reach your 50s, there's a possibility of it changing, and menopause begins to come into effect. A range of serious medical conditions such as heart failure, kidney disease, and stroke are all about high blood pressure; It has been shown that the low-carb keto diet improves blood pressure levels.

7. Increased mass of bones

Aged women are more vulnerable to bone loss, which will ultimately grow into osteoporosis if left uncontrolled and untreated (a medical disorder characterized by weak, fracture-prone bones). Keto removes nutrients that are normally able to interfere with the absorption of calcium. Another advantage of keto is that it, combined with lots of leafy green vegetables that are naturally high in calcium, will improve bone health and density.

8. Weight Sheds

Losing weight has become something close to an impossible challenge as a person gets older. This issue arises from a decline in metabolism rate with age, lack of exercise, healthy activity, and poor diet. However, as the metabolic rate rises and the burning of fats contained in the human body continues to be used, the Keto diet provides the opportunity to combat various problems.

9. Better Sleeping

Sleep disorders such as sleep apnea and insomnia are usually encountered by around 30 years old. An individual must switch to low carb and high fat keto diet to alleviate this and obtain deep sleep at night with additional energy to counteract these disorders.

1.6. What You Can Eat on a Keto Diet

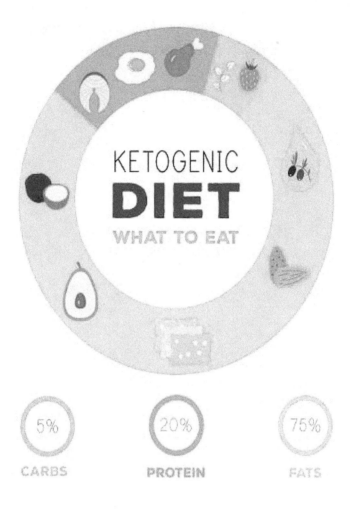

Keto-friendly fats

The largest aspect of a keto diet is to reduce your carb intake to 20-40 net gs per day to attain ketosis. To make sure you're still having the vitamins, minerals, and fiberin your body.

> ➢ Low carb vegetables

> ➢ Low carb fruits

> ➢ Poultry, meat, and eggs

> ➢ Cheese and other dairy products

➢ Seeds and nuts

1. **Poultry, meat, and eggs**: Unprocessed meat is preferred because it contains a minimum amount of carbs with no added carbs.In the keto diet, image findings are essential for eggs. One large egg contains less than 1 gm of carbohydrates, 5 gm of fat, and around 6 gm of protein in terms of nutrition. This nutrient profile is suitable for a ketogenic lifestyle. Egg white protein induces a sensation of fullness and keeps blood sugar levels steady.

2. **Cheese and other dairy products:** pick certain dairy products containing high fats.

3. **Low carb vegetables:** In the keto diet, vegetables that grow above the ground can be included.

4. **Low carb fruit:** the preferred quantity must be mild.

5. **Nut and seeds**: Nuts are a source of fat that is essential. But one must be careful of the volume of their intake.

Keto-friendly beverages: Low carb diets, including certain keto, have a mild diuretic effect, so be sure to drink at least 6 to 8 glasses of water daily, particularly during the induction process, to support your metabolism and normal body functions. The effect of not drinking enough water can be constipation, dizziness, and cravings. Sometimes, to ensure you get enough electrolytes, make sure you add extra salt to your diet. Try sipping your full-sodium broth on your food or adding a little extra salt.Up to 1/2 cup of decaffeinated or regular coffee and tea, herbal tea, sugar-free soy and almond milk, or any of these low-carb drinks are also allowed (without added barley or fruit sugar). Please pay close attention to your beverages, as they're still a big source of hidden sugars and carbohydrates without you knowing.

1.7. What You Can't Eat on the Keto Diet:

1. **Fruits**: are considered high in carbohydrates, so you might assumethat the candy of nature is off-limits on the popular high-fat, low-carbs, so almost all fruits are not permitted to eat in the keto diet.

2. **Legumes:** black beans, kidney beans,etc., are not allowed.

3. **Sweets:**Candy, sweets, cakes, buns, baked goods, tarts, pies, ice cream,cookies, custard, and puddings are not allowed in the keto diet.

4. **Rice:**A meal of no more than three ingredients

5. **Bread:** With a lower concentration of carbohydrates than usual bread

6. **Oatmeal:** With a drop in carb

7. **Pasta:** Getting little more than a recipe of two ingredients

8. **Cooking oil**: Choose from canola oil, soybean oil, grape oil, peanut oil, sesame oil, sunflower oil.

9. **Alcohol:**Keep it as dry as possible if you are going to spring for wine-the bottle should have less than 10g of sugar in its entirety

10. **Bottled condiments:** BBQ sauce, tomato sauce, certain salad dressings, and hot sauces that contain added sugar are bottled condiments that are not allowed.

Chapter 2: Ketogenic diet for women above 50

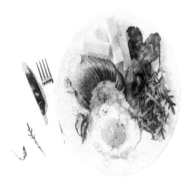

As you shift from adulthood to middle age, many physiological changes occur slowly over time in all body systems. These changes are life events, illness, genetics change, mood swings, and many other factors. According to a scientist, when a person crosses 50, both men and women start to gain 2-lb weight every year. It is most common in women because of their body system, like menopause, causing several hormonal changes in their body, which is weight gain.

Secondly, with aging, the metabolism of your body slows down with increasing age. Still, eating habits do not change, resulting in excess fat accumulation in your body, leading to weight gain. Secondly, your body's metabolism slows down with increasing age, but eating patterns do not change, resulting in excess fat accumulation in your body, leading to weight gain. It also moves forward about age in life, face muscle loss, skin thinning, stomach acidity reduction, and much more. Therefore, with age, by recognizing the variations occurring in the body, you have to start rethinking about eating behaviors to remain fit and safe. Before finalizing your meal schedule, you have to remember your daily workout routine.

People above 50 are less active than young people, so their calorie consumption should be decreased to minimize weight and foods rich in nutrients to remain healthy by consuming different foods to get the right and essential nutrients. Magnesium, omega-3 fatty acids, vitamin D, B12, calcium, iron, and potassium are essential components of older people's diet. Red blood cells responsible for oxygen delivery and brain health are created by vitamin B 12; calcium and vitamin D are essential for bone health. Iron is part of the balanced blood and circulatory system and several other complex benefits. It is also a necessary component of a diet and vitamins, proteins, fibers, and water. With aging, you have to keep the right amount of all these elements in your diet to stay away from diseases and stay healthy because as you get older, the body is unable to maintain the balance of these vitamins and other nutrients, so you can take supplements to support the body.

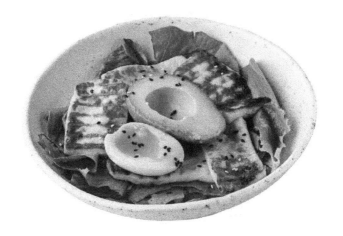

2.1. Sign of aging and loss of nutrients:

1. Change in metabolism

The metabolic rate decreases proportionately with the reduction in total protein tissue. At the very same time, total body fat typically increases with age. Aside from too many calories, lower metabolic rates may also explain this. People tend to increase weight and lose muscle as they get older. It explains why, as you get older, your metabolism will slow down. In general, since they have more body fat, heavier bones, and less body fat than females, men tend to have a faster metabolism.

2. Changes in bone

People, especially women after menopause, lose bone mass or density as they age. Calcium and other minerals are lost to the bones. Bones called vertebrae to make up the spine. A gel-like cushion between each bone is (called a disk)

They can break easily if the bones lose density. As time passes and people get aged, bone density changes. Bones absorb nutrients, water, and minerals during puberty and early adulthood.

3. Digestion Changes

This process often slows down as we age, and this may cause food to pass through the colon more slowly. More water is consumed from food waste as things slow down, which can cause constipation.

Aging may have dramatic effects on the digestive system's functions. Changes in hormone production and an alteration in smell and taste, one of these are decreased appetite. Dysphagia and reflux may result from physiological changes in pharyngeal skills and oesophageal motility. Also, aging can delay the immune system's response to antibodies being produced.

24

4. Sensory alterations

Odor and taste loss affect the food consumption and status of many older adults. It will not be eaten if no food smells or tastes appetizing.Stop eating vegetables until they are mushy. Try to roast or sauté fresh vegetables and toss them with garlic and olive oil until they are lightly fluffy.

Eat variety to meals by choosing foods with different flavored and colors. With dried cranberries and chopped nuts, coat the oatmeal. Add seeds, chickpeas, and crisp vegetables for salads. Start eating small meals more often throughout the day, instead of all three larger meals. It will help to increase your appetite and improve your senses.

5. Constipation and Dehydration

Among the most leading cause of chronic constipation is dehydration. Through your stomach to the large intestine, or colon, the food you consume finds its way. The broad intestine drains water from your food waste if you do not already have enough water in your body.

6. Teeth loss

Poorly fitting dentures will unintentionally alter eating habits due to chewing difficulties. Without important fresh fruits and vegetables, the result may be a sluggish, low-fiberdiet.As a way of preventing or slowing down the aging process, various items are advertised. Yet, there is no hard scientific evidence to prove that all these goods are healthy.

Instead, gerontologists (aging experts) suggest that people focus on staying healthy and well so that they can enjoy their favorite hobbies in middle age and beyond. Eating a balanced diet, which contains all the necessary nutrients for health, is a big part of a healthy lifestyle. Here are the main variables that, as you age, influence your nutritional health.

2.2. Solutions

1. Needs for Calories

Our resting metabolic rate decreases as we grow older. It can lead to undesirable weight gain, which can increase the risk of some chronic diseases. As we age, this drop in metabolic rate is linked to the loss of lean body mass. To assist in reducing this effect:Increase your physical activity so that more calories are consumed.To strengthen your muscles and gain muscle mass, which increases your metabolic rate, start resistance training—incorporating whole grains, fruits and vegetables, lean protein, and non-fat or low-fat dairy improves your diet's consistency.

2. Proteins

For tissue development, repair, and maintenance, protein is essential. It's necessary to eat an adequate amount of protein each day, despite the need for fewer calories as we age. 45 to 60 gs are required by the average adult. Choose high-quality protein foods.

3. Dental health

Eighty percent of adult Americans are reported to have periodontal disease. Good practices in dental hygiene can help prevent it. As a result, foods such as fresh fruits, vegetables, and meat can be avoided. For the prevention of periodontal disease:

- Have dental tests and cleanings on an annual basis.
- During meals or after eating high-sugar food, brush your teeth.
- Floss periodically.

4. Taste

Sometimes, the senses of taste and smell are dulled by the aging process. Your sense of taste can also change with smoking and certain drugs. The protection of taste and smell:Keep hydrated; to completely taste the food, adequate saliva is required.

- Refrain from overusing the saltshaker.
- To boost the taste of food, use herbs and spices.

5. Antioxidant agents

There is no conclusive evidence that antioxidant supplements such as vitamin C or E can help prevent or postpone the aging process by avoiding chronic diseases. In reality, consuming foods rich in antioxidants (whole grains, fruits, and vegetables) and not taking supplements is beneficial. In your diet, include more of these

- To the Almonds
- Peppers from the Bell (especially red and orange)
- Blueberry
- Dark green vegetables with leaves
- Strawberry
- Tomatoes and Tomatoes

5. Vitamin D and Calcium

The bulk of the calcium in our bodies is in our bones. This mineral is needed for the nervous system's proper function, muscle contractions, and blood clotting. For the prevention and treatment of osteoporosis, sufficient calcium intake is crucial; vitamin D is important for calcium absorption. Dairy foods are also the best calcium source because the body can quickly absorb calcium in them.

The optimum amount of calcium for healthy adults is discussed by experts. Try to get all your calcium from food sources where possible. Except for fortified dairy products, vitamin D is not commonly present in foods. So you may need a supplement to take it. The body produces vitamin D from sunlight exposure, but people in northern climates do not get sufficient sun exposure to make adequate quantities of the vitamin in the winter. The new vitamin D intake guidelines suggest 600 IU for adults 19 to 70 years of age and 800 IU for those over 70.

6. Nutritional Supplements

If a person has a vitamin or mineral deficiency, health care practitioners usually do not prescribe dietary supplements. More research demonstrates that the best source of nutrients is food, not tablets or commercial beverages. Keep yourself in mind:

More is not necessarily better with vitamins; a multivitamin and mineral supplement should be everything you need to compensate for any shortfalls in your diet.

When eating a balanced diet, vitamin D and, in some cases, calcium is the only nutrients you need. There is insufficient evidence to encourage nutritional supplements with antioxidants.

7. Water

Sometimes, water is a forgotten nutrient. But for almost all bodily functions, having enough fluid is important. Approximately 1.5 to 2 liters or 48 to 64 ounces of fluid per day is required by healthy adults. As we age, the sense of thirst decreases, which leaves us susceptible to dehydration. Focus on non-diuretic beverages, such as decaffeinated foods, fruit juices, non-fat or low-fat milk, and water, of course.

All these things come in a keto diet plan

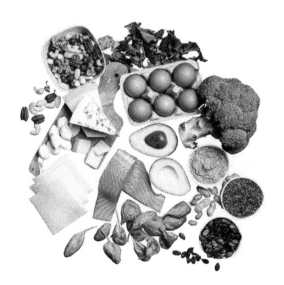

2.3. Is the keto diet good for women over 50?

One factor that never determines whether or notketo is right for you, but before assuming that keto is right for you, there are many factors involved.

Suppose you don't suffer from any significant health problems; in that case, a ketogenic diet will quench an enormous advantage, more precisely losing weight and getting rid of excess fat and obesity, the root cause of many. When eating vegetables, meat, and carbs, one must maintain equilibrium, as required. It is not easy to adapt and adhere to a ketogenic diet, as shown by many studies, so the best technique is to follow the balanced diet that suits you best and then stick to it. It is usually good to try new stuff, but one must think thousands of times before trying something new where there is a health danger.

The ketogenic diet is so genuine and successful that its consumers have consistently recorded its miraculous potency. Women record falling 11 lbs in seven days, up to 49 lbs in eight weeks, and almost 200+ lbs to their full limit so far, including in some instances, as reported.

2.4. How to start keto for women over 50

Keto is a simple diet, high carb diet to eating 50 gs of carbs or less per day is not always easy. It is just a mere difference in consumption and requires an adaptation in lifestyle that only exaggerates how much of a commitment this diet is. However, these minor changes deliver brilliant results and, in effect, are only the stepping stones to a healthier and sustainable life as it is guaranteed that these minuscule amendments will have a long-term effect not just physically but mentally too. Though at first, itmay seem intimidating, it does get much easier and understandable.

By following these instructions, make the transition into low carb keto dieting simpler.

1. Have a scheduled plan diet:

Keto is so specific from other diets that you cannot just jump in without doing your homework. Pick a start date and give yourself time to learn the ins and outs of low-carb dieting.

Learn more about what you can and can't eat. Spend this time gathering some low-carb instruments that may be useful, such as meal plans and recipes.

Also, tell your friends and family that you will 'go keto' and that your diet is about to change. Inform them to be supportive and agree that you won't eat bread, rice, pasta, etc.

2. Clear the unnecessary carbs out of your cupboards

Clean out any non-keto foods from your kitchen and refrigerator shortly before you begin your keto diet. You may think you can avoid temptation and not consume it, but the fact is that if you have easy access to high-carb foods, you are more likely to violate your diet.

However, don'teat any of these foods. The more carbohydrates you ingest, the harder and slower the transition to ketosis will be.

3. Using an app for food monitoring

Successful dieting with keto means restricting the consumption of carb to 50 gs a day or less. Using a food tracking app is the simplest and easiest way to lose weight and be your diet plan. Effective choices include good options,

It is an easy-to-use macro tracker; your meals can be fine-tuned to get the right carbohydrates, protein, and fat in your diet.

4. Realize that the first two weeks are the worst,

It's not always easy to get a keto, particularly for the first two weeks. Your body takes time to use all its onboard carb stores and instead make the transition to using ketones for energy. During this time, certain individuals experience adverse side effects, which as keto flu.

Although it is not serious and certainly you can feel unwell once the body completely reaches ketosis.

Popular symptoms of keto flu include:

- Headache
- Nausea
- Constipation
- Sleeplessness
- Fruity-odorous breath
- Increase in urination
- Tiredness
- Swings of mood
- Cravings

You are well on the way to being a machine for fat-burning. Your symptoms will fade soon, and they will fully pass within 1-2 weeks. Often, after they leave, and unless you cheat on your diet, only once can you ever suffer keto flu.

5. Don't cheat at all

Many diets allow you to take days off and even cheat by eating unhealthy foods from time to time. The keto diet is not either of those diets If you cheat on keto by consuming carbohydrates, you can push yourself out of ketosis to have to go through another bout of keto flu to get back on track.

Don't be tempted to trick keto. Long story short, it's just not worth it. Alternatively, in some types of therapy, reward your healthy eating habits. It's a nice idea to go to the movies, buy a new fitness suite, or treat yourself to a massage or beauty treatment. High carb food treats are not found in the ketogenic diet.

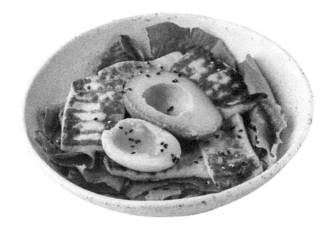

6. Think of using some well-picked supplements

Although you don't have to use supplements on the keto diet, for women over 50, they can make things simpler. Great choices include:

7. Ketones exogenous

Ketones from an external source are exogenous ketones. Taking exogenous ketone supplements will speed up burning fat, give you energy, keep your mind calm, and help alleviate many symptoms of keto flu. As drink blends and in capsules, exogenous ketones are available.

8. Triglycerides of the medium-chain

These specific fats are quickly and easily converted by MCTs, for short, into ketones. More ketones mean better fat burning and weight loss, more control, and fewerketo flu symptoms.

MCT supplements are used to make palm or coconut oil. However, coconut oil is the best and is also the most environmentally conscious choice. There are MCTs available as oils or in easy-to-mix powder form.

9. Electrolytes

In your urine, electrolytes are minerals that are excreted and even lost when you sweat.The keto diet raises urine production, which could mean that your body begins to run low on these vital substances. Symptoms of low electrolyte levels include headaches and muscle cramps. Electrolyte supplements supplement absent nutrients that can help prevent a number of symptoms of keto flu.

10. Treat keto as a way of life, not just a diet.

Most people think about a new diet; they just want it to be practiced for a few weeks. They figure that they will get through it until they have lost some weight and then go back to their previous eating habits. It eventually leads to weight loss, dubbed yoyo dieting by experts, followed by weight recovery. You will get even better keto outcomes if you accept low-carb dieting as a lifestyle choice and not a short-term fix. That way, you're not only going to lose weight, but you're also going to keep it off for good. Most of the benefits listed earlier in this chapter only refer to dieting on a low-carb basis. If you break your diet, lower blood pressure, improved cardiovascular health, reduced inflammation, and better bone health, you can say goodbye to such factors. If you break your diet, lower blood pressure, improved cardiovascular health, reduced inflammation, and better bone health, you can say goodbye to such factors. Keto is perfect for weight loss in your 50s, but it can be so much more than that as well. It can have a profound and substantial effect on any aspect of your welfare. After a few weeks or months, by reaching and quitting keto, do not give away those advantages. Instead, make a long-term commitment to low-carb diets. You will love the result if you do.

2.5. What makes keto-diet so powerful?

A ketogenic diet speeds up our body's metabolic response, which helps metabolically transform our body. If we do a detailed analysis, it will be discovered that one is persuaded to abstain from eating carbohydrates to the degree that ketosis is caused in one's body by following a keto diet. Several medical doctors reported that those patients who religiously followed the keto diet increased their fat-burning process by almost 900 percent. As a consequence, the hollowness caused by the internal burning of the fat causes them to shrink.

Another benefit of the keto diet is that it changes the human body's metabolism, accelerating its normal metabolism rate to about ten times. In deciding the metabolic rate, muscle tissues are used. A short study was carried out at a university in southern California, which demonstrated that they lose muscle tissue annually when women leap over 30 years of age. Besides, this phenomenon brings speed in tandem with time, some of them losing a substantial 20 percent of their muscles as they leap over the 60s, resulting in their metabolism slowing down. This lack of muscles causes a large chunk of their body mass, No need to worry because a keto diet is full of protein and healthy fats that trigger the revival of these missing muscles and provides them with an alternative. Thus, reviving metabolism and helping them sustain their healthy speed result from which, women will not suffer mass and health loss when they grow old.

Expediting metabolism is the key advantage that can be extracted from the keto diet. Still, certain secondary advantages of the keto diet include nourishing our body with satiety hormones and the like. Besides, many individuals feel dissatisfied adopting the diet plan in addition to providing a multitude of benefits. Most of them do not abstain from eating tasty items that catch their attention with carbohydrates. It is normally difficult to limit yourself from eating favorite meals and eating only the exact quantity of proteins, fats measured and carefully reduce the number of carbohydrates to 5 percent in our diet when consuming the number of meals three times a day. Many keto dieters claim that before getting completely beneficial from the keto diet, determining the diet plan requires math at a severely intimidating stage. This drastic calculation also results in a lack of motivation and satisfaction when following the diet, thereby leading most dieters to abandon their diet plan. However, as successful as keto is, many women are struggling with the diet. Many weight loss methods are too difficult to sustain long enough to build new behaviors, doctors explain. By decreasing carbohydrates, proteins, and fats to 5%, 25%, and 70%, respectively, the initial version of the keto diet asks to restrict macronutrients, and this measurement is very tiring and a hassle for most people, resulting in missing this calorie count most of the time

Fortunately, when preparing the diet, keto dieters have come across another way to get rid of the laborious math. The projected concept rests on keeping the diet plan easy in which one can bypass the traditional proposed keto diet and can forge their diet plan, and instructions on the diet plan could be obtained to help in this regard.

The Keto diet helps you get thin in no time, but it also helps minimize heart diseases. The keto diet also helps preserve the balance of cholesterol, preventing the usual defense and reversal of diabetes from artery damage three times. Besides, it is also beneficial to the brain because several repeated studies have shown that it significantly improves the dieter's memory and decreases arthritis discomfort.

2.6. A common problem

They envelop their frustrating tales and worst experience when trying to follow the keto diet, as reported by the number of physicians during the study that many patients give them emails. Doctors have often received an email from people who complained about the diet's ineffectiveness when saying they had diligently followed the diet plan. Still, sadly, however, they do not lose weight. Despite their urine showing that they are undergoing ketosis, some individuals complained that they are gaining weight instead of losing weight, causing them further anger. Let me clarify one explanation for this diet's ineffectiveness for women aged between 40 and 50 years. Do not worry if you are suffering from this anomaly because you are not alone. During the 1940s, many women in the United Kingdom and the United States had menopause. It does not matter which diet you adopt during this transition period; you will be gaining weight.

But it is advised that they should not worry, the best top ten tips for such individuals are carefully advised mentioned below but note if one out of many tips does not prove successful but must try because the last tip will be a practical one.

- **Get the proper quantity of protein**

Protein must be eaten to a moderate sustainable extent for weight loss. Moreover, It is proven by female physicians that women typically eat more protein than male partners; If a woman and her husband eat a protein-containing steak, she must consume it in more quantities than his husband.

Doctors had put forth an idea to tackle the confusing task of gcounting. A solution was A 'Mindful Week,' which was proposed by them. It requires the interpretation of the hunger and fullness principle. Doctors say that most of the Sapiens do not understand the basic notionand distinction between hunger and fullness. Discussing the real problem, doctors say that most women are not suffering because of menopause but because of their lack of appetite andfulfillment.

In the meantime, doctors' approach is limited to women experiencing menopause and is accessible to any woman over 30 who has decided to lose weight and improve health. Coming to a point, what is the week of mindfulness? It is a time commitment task during which, before recognizing that what is enough for her exceeds her original requirement, one has toobserve her hunger and fullness closely.

Let us consider a brief example of this method. Try eating two loaves of bread at breakfast, but you'll eat one instead of two today. After twenty mins, you will find either hungry or need one more leaf to kill your hunger. You will come to know the right amount of food to satisfy your appetite, following the same routine and sagaciously observing yourself. That will help you stop eating, which normally leads to gaining weight. But to have a healthy body with strong muscles, one should bear in mind that proteins are a vital part of a diet, so be very careful when cutting your protein intake.

- **Don't eat too much fat**

Since the keto diet is focused on high fats and low carbohydrates, for those who love to eat fats, this low carb keto diet is cheerful because it is included in every meal. Simultaneously, since fat is highly concentrated in the keto diet, one must abstain from consuming too much fat. According to experts, if you want to get rid of your weight, you must burn the body's fat. On the contrary, if one is persistent through his keto diet in eating fat and striving to burn fats accumulated in one's body, all his struggles will be wasted. Taking fats through the keto diet will replace those burned by the challenging efforts of one.

Doctors typically show that every new keto dieter is addicted to eating many carbohydrates in glucose, coffee, and whipping cream before adopting the keto diet. He recommended that they substitute these carbohydrates with high fats, and once they are completely removed from carbohydrates, they are then recommended to limit the fat limit. Due to its realistic use, the technique is proposed. It is much harder to get rid of the addictiveness of carbohydrates compared to that of fats. So it becomes easier for them to turn their diet from fat to keto-friendly food products without putting much effort when a person stops eating carbohydrates. Besides, a person typically begins to enjoy keto diet plans, producing more pleasant results.

When one gets rid of eating carbs' addictiveness and yet experiences a halt in weight loss, the volume of fat consumption must be considered. One will certainly figure out the real loophole causing this weight loss stall by analyzing its fat intake. In small steps, one must slowly cut back a min of coffee to stay relaxed while attempting to cut back some of the fat in one's diet to break the stall. In several situations, doctors remember that people complain about losing weight from the stall while saying that they strictly observe the keto diet but cannot produce the desired results. When doctors asked them to present their diet plan, which they were pursuing, it was discovered that by overdosing on coffee and whipped cream whose main constituent is fat, they were eating an abundance of fat. After recognizing their diet strategies, their respective doctor is recommended to cut back some of the fat they eat in coffee and whooping to break this stall and achieve the desired outcomes.

The good thing is that this technique does not place a total restriction on fat intake, but it only involves weight reduction by cutting fat before the stall breaks. The weight soon reaches the optimal amount; one can raise fat intake to whatever level one wants to eat.

- **Pay attention to the carb creep**

When an individual is thoroughly following the low carb, high fat keto diet, special care must be taken to avoid carbs' consumption. Carbs are often found in sauces, vegetables, nut snacks, and condiments. Often, carbohydrates will reach your diet without knowing by eating carelessly, so there is a huge risk of consuming carbs through sauces, fruits, nut snacks, and seasonings, which must be avoided by eating carefully.

Time and again, the same lesson is cited to emphasize the main factor to which people typically do not pay much attention, leading them to lose the efficacy of the keto diet. It is suggested that you need to revisit your current diet at the drop of a hat. There may be an abundance of carbs that have become unnoticeably part of your meal.

Nuts such as cashews and pistachios are difficult to overeat while having enough carbohydrates to lead to weight-loss stalling. Like, for example, pistachios, which contain around 21 gs of carbohydrates. Those people who avoid insulin can experience a ketosis stall for about three weeks if they eat food-containing carbohydrates. The dieter would certainly find a good outcome if the keto dieter carefully kept the amount of carbohydrate intake below 20 gs.

- **Cut the Alcohol Out**

Alcohol lovers are experiencing ketosis, and they are persuaded that they should have a few bottles of weekly wine time and time again following a low carb diet plan. But for them, it is bad news that alcohol overconsumption may lead to a weight-loss stall. However, if one comes to know that, while thoroughly pursuing one's keto diet schedule, one is not losing weight, one should doubt that alcohol intake is this stall. It would be wise to cut back all wine intake before the ketosis started again if caught in such a situation.

- **Stop eating sweets**

Many individuals are likely to use artificial flavors to feel relaxed when eating the keto diet. Even if these sweeteners, such as sucralose or aspartame, give one's meal the perfect taste, it may be equally disadvantageous for those who observe the keto diet. Typically, therefore, experts prohibit keto dieters from adding sweeteners to their diets. Experts do not clarify why one should avoid using sweeteners because of a lack of studies on this topic, but most agree with the decision.People who cut sweeteners from their diet lose weight easily.

- **Get enough sleep**

A proper night's sleep plummets with tension and cortisol. Cortisol is a stress hormone that induces an increase in abdominal fat when elevated. Owing to night sweats and hot flashes, women suffering from menopause still face a condition in which their sleeping routine is ruined. It is recommended for these women, who are involved in weight loss, to keep their primary focus on following their proper sleeping routine while going through the menopause era, keeping all stresses at bay. A bad sleeping pattern causes cortisol, a stress hormone linked to abdominal fat, while increasing the human body's weight.

For better sleep, tips include:

- ➢ Limit caffeine intake and stop drinking coffee

- ➢ Spend some time in the sunlight.

- ➢ Using eyeshades and earplugs to wear

- ➢ Try to restrict screen time before reaching the bed to stop the blue light (or if possible, use glasses that blocks blue light)

- ➢ Craft a suitable sleeping schedule and religiously execute it.

- ➢ It must be cool and dark in the sleeping room.

- ➢ Stop drinking before reaching the bed.

- • Stress Reduction

Weaning off all sorts of stresses that you are dealing with is vital. Stress often puts one's mental and physical health at an adverse risk.

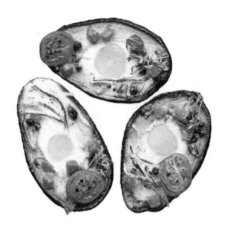

Below is a range of recipes recommended by nutritionists and experts to help get your diet started. Most require normal 'around the house' items to help get your breakfast, lunch, and dinner in full swing,

1) Bacon Breakfast Biscuit

Ingredients:

> 6 bacon slices (chopped).

> 3 large eggs

> 1 cup cheddar cheese (grated)

> 1 cup onion (chopped)

> 1 cup green peppers (chopped)

> ¾ cup almond flour

> 1 tsp baking powder

43

- ➤ ½ tsp salt
- ➤ ½ tsp pepper
- ➤ Cooking spray

Instructions:

1. Preheat the oven to 375 degrees C.

2. Spray the cooking spray with a large frying pan and fry the bacon until it is crisp and browned. Add the onions and peppers, cut the bacon and fry until tender.

3. Mix the almond flour, baking powder, salt, and pepper in a bowl until well mixed.

4. Whisk the eggs in a separate bowl and add half a cup of the cheese; add the mixture of eggs to the flour mixture and blend until well combined; whisk in the cooked bacon.

5. Line a baking tray with greaseproof paper; spoon to flatten 12 individual round biscuits slightly with the back of a spoon on the sticky mixture.

6. Sprinkle the remaining cheese over it and bake for 10 mins.

Nutritional Information:

- ➤ Total servings - 12 Per serving: (1 biscuit)
- ➤ Fat: 33g
- ➤ Carbohydrates: 4g
- ➤ Protein: 31g
- ➤ Calories: 451

2) Egg & Goats Cheese Medley

Ingredients:

- ➤ 8 large eggs
- ➤ 1 tomato (chopped)

- ➢ 2 oz goats' cheese
- ➢ 2 tbsp water
- ➢ ¼ cup mixed fresh herbs (chopped)
- ➢ 1 tbsp butter
- ➢ ½ tsp salt
- ➢ ¼ tsp black pepper

Instructions:

1. Whisk the eggs, salt, pepper, and water together.

2. Heat the butter in a large frying pan, add the egg mixture and cook for 2-3 mins, mix in the tomatoes and remove from the heat.

3. Fold the goat's cheese and herbs together.

Nutritional Information:

- ➢ Total servings - 4 Per serving
- ➢ Fat: 10g
- ➢ Carbohydrates: 2g
- ➢ Protein: 15g
- ➢ Calories: 249

3) Nutty Cottage Cheese Fruit Mingle

Ingredients:

- ➢ ¾ cup cottage cheese
- ➢ ¼ cup frozen mixed berries
- ➢ 3 tbsp walnuts (chopped)
- ➢ 1 tsp flaxseed oil
- ➢ 1 tsp chia seeds.

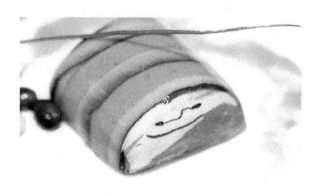

➢

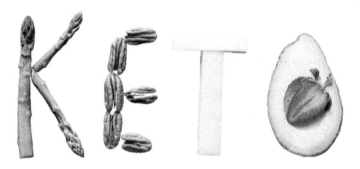

Instructions:

1. In a bowl, add the cottage cheese and drizzle it with flaxseed oil.

2. Sprinkle with the chia seeds and finish with walnuts and mixed berries.

Nutritional Information:

- ➢ Total servings - 1 Per serving
- ➢ Fat: 23g
- ➢ Carbohydrates: 11g
- ➢ Protein: 19g
- ➢ Calories: 312

4) Egg & Bacon Sandwich Twist

Ingredients:

- ➢ 4 bacon slices
- ➢ 3 large eggs
- ➢ 1 tomato (chopped)
- ➢ 1 spring onion (chopped)
- ➢ ¾ cup mozzarella
- ➢ ¾ cup cheddar cheese
- ➢ Cooking spray

Instructions:

1. Preheat the oven at 400 and line a baking tray with parchment paper.

2. Mix the cheese and spread it on the tray evenly, creating a circle—Bake for approximately 5 mins.

3. Spray with a cooking spray on a frying pan, fry the bacon until crispy and remove from the pan. Spray and scramble the eggs with a little more cooking spray.

4. On one half of the cheese circle, put the bacon and eggs: sprinkle on the tomato and onion.

5. Over the bacon and eggs, fold the cheese circle in half, press down firmly, and bake for 5 mins.

Nutritional Information:

- ➢ Total servings - 2 Per serving:
- ➢ Fat: 35g
- ➢ Carbohydrates: 5g
- ➢ Protein: 33g
- ➢ Calories: 445

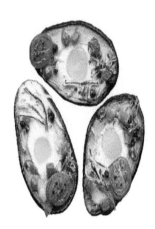

5) Chorizo & Egg Breakfast Buns

Ingredients:

- ➢ 12 eggs
- ➢ 6 oz cheddar cheese (grated)
- ➢ 5 oz chorizo (chopped)
- ➢ 2 spring onions (chopped)
- ➢ Salt and pepper

> ➢ Cooking spray

Instructions:

1. Preheat the oven to 350 and grease a large muffin tray.

2. Add the chorizo and onions to the bottom of each hole in the muffin tray.

3. Whisk the eggs, cheese, salt, and pepper together; pour the onions and chorizo on top.

4. Bake until done, for approximately 20-25 mins.

Nutritional information:

> ➢ Total servings - 6 Per serving: (2 buns)
> ➢ Fat: 27g
> ➢ Carbohydrates: 2g
> ➢ Protein: 23g
> ➢ Calories: 335

6) Loaded Avocado

Ingredients:

> ➢ 4 eggs
> ➢ 4 cherry tomatoes (chopped)
> ➢ 6 oz bacon (chopped)
> ➢ 2 avocados
> ➢ Cooking spray

Instructions:

1. Preheat the oven to 375.

2. Spray cooking spray onto a frying pan and fry the bacon until crispy.

3. Cut the avocados, remove the stone; to fit an egg, and scoop out enough flesh.

4. On a baking tray, put the avocados and crack an egg in each hole. Sprinkle the tomatoes over the eggs along with the bacon.

5. Bake for 20 mins until the eggs are cooked thoroughly.

Nutritional Information:

- ➢ Total servings - 2 Per serving:
- ➢ Fat: 73g
- ➢ Carbohydrates: 6g
- ➢ Protein: 25g
- ➢ Calories: 803

7) Coconut & Blueberry Porridge

Ingredients:

- ➢ 1 large egg
- ➢ ¼ cup blueberries
- ➢ 1 oz butter
- ➢ 1 tbsp coconut flour
- ➢ 4 tbsp coconut cream
- ➢ 1 pinch psyllium husk powder

Instructions:

1. In a cup, whisk the egg and stir in the psyllium husk and coconut flour.

2. Melt the butter on low heat and add the coconut milk. Combine the egg mixture slowly until it becomes thick and fluffy.

3. Add the blueberries.

Nutritional Information:

- ➢ Total servings - 1 Per serving:

- ➢ Fat: 50g
- ➢ Carbohydrates: 4g
- ➢ Protein: 10g
- ➢ Calories: 488

8) Sweet & Spicy Stuffed Peppers

Ingredients:

- ➢ 8 ounces Cream cheese
- ➢ 8 mini bell peppers
- ➢ 1 ounce's chorizo (chopped)
- ➢ 2 tbsp Olive oil for
- ➢ 1/2 tbsp Chipotle paste

Instructions:

1.Mix all ingredients until well combined.

2. Put the mixture of spoons into peppers.

Nutrition facts:

- ➢ Total servings - 4 Per serving
- ➢ Fat: 31
- ➢ Carbohydrates: 8g
- ➢ Protein: 8g
- ➢ Calories: 343

9) Cheesy Cauliflower Combo

Ingredients:

- ➢ Cauliflower 28 ounces (chopped)
- ➢ Broccoli 16 ounces (chopped)
- ➢ Cheddar cheese 8 ounces (grated)

- ➤ Cream cheese of 7 ounces
- ➤ 1 cup of cream thick
- ➤ Two ounces of butter
- ➤ 2 Tsp of powdered garlic

Instructions:

1.Boil the broccoli in a large saucepan until thoroughly cooked and tender.

2. Strain and leave the broccoli in a saucepan; add cream cheese, thick cream, butter, and powdered garlic.

3. Purée until smooth and creamy using a blender

4. Grease a large baking platter and add florets of cauliflower.

5. Pour over a mixture of creamy broccoli and top with cheese.

6. Cook until the cauliflower is tender and the cheese is golden, for 40-45 mins.

Nutrition Facts:

- ➤ Total servings - 6 Per serving
- ➤ Fat: 45g
- ➤ Carbohydrates: 11g
- ➤ Protein: 18g
- ➤ Calories: 5133

10) Avocado &Chili Crab Salad

Ingredients:

- ➤ 12 ounces of meat from crab (canned)
- ➤ 4 eggs of large size (boiled)

- ➤ 2 avocados
- ➤ 2 ounces baby Spinach
- ➤ 2 tbsps Olive oil
- ➤ 1/2 cup Mayonnaise
- ➤ 1/2 cup of cottage cheese.
- ➤ 1/2 tbsps of chili flakes

Instructions:

1.Slice the avocados and chop the boiled eggs into halves.

2. Drain the meat from the crab and stir in the chili flakes.

3. Place the eggs, avocado, mayonnaise, cottage cheese, crab meat, and spinach on a plate.

4. Drizzle the spinach with olive oil.

Nutritional details:

- ➤ Total Portions - 2 Per Portion
- ➤ Fat: 98g Fat:
- ➤ Carbohydrates: 7g
- ➤ 44g Protein
- ➤ 1097 Calories

11) Cheeky Cheesy Chips

Ingredients:

- ➤ Cheddar cheese 8 ounces (grated)
- ➤ Cheddar cheese 8 ounces (grated)
- ➤ Chili flakes with 1/2 tsp
- ➤ 1/2 tsp of paprika

Instructions:

1.Preheat the oven to 400.

2. Line a parchment paper baking tray and a cheese spoon into separate piles.

3. Sprinkle chili flakes and paprika with cheese piles and bake until fully melted and golden for 10 mins.

4. Allow to cool down.

Nutritional Information:

- ➢ Total servings - 4 Per serving
- ➢ Fat: 22g
- ➢ Carbohydrates: 2g
- ➢ Protein: 12g
- ➢ Calories: 229

12) Bacon & Halloumi Sausages

Ingredients:

- ➢ 8-ounce halloumi
- ➢ 6 ounces Bacon

Instructions:

1. Preheat the oven to 425.
2. Cut the halloumi into 10 chunks and wrap around each chunk with a slice of bacon.
3. Bake for 15-20 mins, turning until cooked through and golden brown occasionally.

Nutritional Information:

- ➢ Total servings - 2 Per serving
- ➢ Fat: 63g
- ➢ Carbohydrates: 4g
- ➢ Protein: 33g
- ➢ Calories: 703

13) Pork in Garlic & Red Wine

Ingredients:

- Pork shoulder of 48 ounce
- 6 cloves of garlic
- 6 leaves of Iceberg lettuce
- 2 onions of red
- 3/4 cup of red wine
- 1/2 cup of olive oil
- 2 tbsps of cilantro (finely chopped)
- Salt of 1/2 tsp
- Ground cinnamon with 2 tsps
- 2 black pepper tsp
- Dried thyme with 2 tsps

Instructions:

1. Preheat the stove to 250.
2. Slice the onions into thin wedges and cut the garlic in half.
3. Add the remaining marinating ingredients. In a large ziplock bag, put the pork shoulder and pour in the marinade.
4. Seal the bag and put it in a big dish overnight, in refrigerate.
5. Place the pork and marinade in a large oven-proof dish, cover with a close-fitting lid.
6. Bake for 6-7 hours in the lower portion of the oven.
7. Pork is exceptionally tender to serve on top of lettuce leaves and take apart.

Nutritional Information:

- ➢ Total servings - 4 Per serving
- ➢ Fat: 92g
- ➢ Carbohydrates:11g
- ➢ Protein: 63g
- ➢ Calories: 1141

14) Pan-Seared Pork & Pepper

Ingredients:

- ➢ 10-ounce pork (cut into strips)
- ➢ 4-ounce butter
- ➢ 1 red pepper (chopped)
- ➢ 1 yellow pepper (chopped)
- ➢ 1 red onion (sliced)
- ➢ 1 tsp chili paste.

Instructions:

1. Heat butter in a pan on high heat and brown pork for 3 mins.
2. Add in remaining ingredients and fry until thoroughly cooked.

Nutritional Information:

- ➢ Total servings - 2 Per serving
- ➢ Fat: 79g
- ➢ Carbohydrates: 4g
- ➢ Protein: 29g
- ➢ Calories: 840

15) Zucchini & Sausage Stew

Ingredients:

- ➢ 16 ounces sausage
- ➢ Mozzarella 8 ounces (grated)
- ➢ Marinara sauce with 7 ounces
- ➢ 6 ounces of bacon (chopped)
- ➢ Cream cheese of 4 ounce
- ➢ 4 ounces of parmesan (grated)
- ➢ Two zucchinis (grated)
- ➢ For 2 eggs
- ➢ 1 of onions (finely chopped).

Instructions:

1. Preheat the oven to 400.
2. Mix until well combined: zucchinis, cream cheese, milk, parmesan, and 4 oz mozzarella.
3. For 18-20 mins, pour the mixture into an oven-proof dish and bake.
4. Cook the onions, sausage, and bacon in a large frying pan until cooked through.
5. Take the zucchini from the oven, spread it over the marinara sauce, and top it with the sausage mixture.
6. Top and bake for an additional 15 mins with the remaining mozzarella.

Nutritional Information:

- ➢ Total servings - 6 Per serving
- ➢ Fat: 59g
- ➢ Carbohydrates: 8g
- ➢ Protein: 33g

> Calories: 693

16) Mediterranean Meatballs & Mozzarella

Ingredients:

> 16 ounces of beef mince.

> 14 ounces of tomatoes whole (canned)

> Spinach 7 ounces

> Mozzarella for 5 ounces

> Two ounces of butter

> ounces of parmesan (grated)

> For 1 egg

> Olive oil 3 tbsps

> tbsps of chives (chopped)

> 1 tsp salt

> 1 tsp of powdered garlic

> Onion powder of 1/2 tbsp

> Dried basil 1/2 tsp

> Black pepper, 1/2 tsp

Instructions

1. Mix the beef, parmesan, egg, and spices in a large bowl until well combined.

2. Make the blend into meatballs of walnut size.

3. In a frying pan, heat the oil and fry the meatballs until cooked and browned.

4. Turn down the heat and add the chives and tomatoes.

5. Allow 15-20 mins to simmer.

6. Melt the butter and fry the spinach for 2 mins in a separate frying pan and add to the meatballs.

7. On a serving plate, put the meatballs, tear up the mozzarella, and drip over the meatballs.

Nutritional Information:

➢ Total servings - 4 Per serving

➢ Fat: 51g

➢ Carbohydrates: 4g

➢ Protein: 40g

➢ Calories: 626

17) Salmon & Pistachio Hot Pot

Ingredients:

➢ 15-ounce fillets of salmon

➢ 10 ounces of cherry tomatoes

➢ 1/2 cup of green olives (pitted & chopped)

➢ 1/3 cup of pistachio nuts (chopped)

➢ 1/4 cup of olive oil

➢ 1/4 cup of fresh dill (chopped)

Instructions:

1. Preheat the oven to 350.

2. Mix the olives and pistachios along with a splash of olive oil until well blended.

3. In an oven-proof bowl, put the salmon fillets and spread the olive mixture around the dish. Place the tomatoes in a separate oven-proof dish and cover with olive oil.

4. Bake both for 15 mins and sprinkle them with dill until thoroughly cooked.

Nutritional Information:

- ➢ Total servings - 2 Per serving
- ➢ Fat: 69g
- ➢ Carbohydrates: 7g
- ➢ Protein: 48g
- ➢ Calories: 844

18) Chicken with Onion Mayo

Ingredients:

- ➢ 16-ounce breast of chicken
- ➢ 7 ounces of green cabbage (chopped)
- ➢ 1/2 cup of mayonnaise
- ➢ 1/2 of red onion (finely sliced)
- ➢ 1 tbsp Olive oil
- ➢ Spray for cooking.

Instructions:

1. Cook the chicken until thoroughly cooked in a large frying pan sprinkled with cooking spray. Mix the onions and mayonnaise.
2. Place the chopped cabbage and drizzle with olive oil in the middle of the serving plate.
3. Place the chicken on top of the cabbage gently and put onion mayonnaise on the side.

Nutritional Information:

- ➢ Total servings - 2 Per serving
- ➢ Fat: 93g
- ➢ Carbohydrates: 7g
- ➢ Protein: 47g

> Calories: 1039

19) Beef & Tomato Pie

Ingredients:

> A minced beef of 14 ounces

> 9 ounces of cherry tomatoes (halved)

> 3 onions chopped)

> 3 carrots (chopped)

> 3 cloves of garlic (grated)

> 1/2 head of cauliflower (cut into florets)

> 1/4 cup of olive oil.

Instructions:

1. Preheat the furnace to 350.

2. Boil the water in a wide pan and add the cauliflower; cook until tender.

3. In a frying pan, add a little olive oil and cook until the carrots, onion, and garlic are cooked through.

4. Add the minced beef to the frying pan and cook until the tomatoes are browned.

5. Pour the mixture of beef into an oven-proof dish.

6. Add cauliflower and a little olive oil in a bowl, mash cauliflower until creamy and smooth. Spoon the cauliflower mixture over the beef and bake until golden brown for 20 mins.

Nutritional Information:

> Total servings - 6 Per serving

> Fat: 20g

> Carbohydrates: 9g

➢ Protein: 15g

➢ Calories: 270

20) Aromatic Spinach & Cheese Curry

Ingredients:

➢ Spinach of 14 ounces

➢ 7 ounces halloumi (cubed)

➢ Curry paste of 3 tbsps

➢ Olive oil for 2 tbsps

➢ 1 tbsp of cumin seed

➢ 1 slice of black pepper.

Instructions:

1. Mix the olive oil and curry paste in a large bowl; stir in the cubed halloumi.

2. Pour the mixture into a frying pan and cook until the cheese starts to melt for 5-6 mins. Toast the cumin seeds in a separate frying pan until they start to smoke; add some olive oil and spinach, fry until cooked, and season with pepper.

3. Place the spinach and top with cheese on a serving plate.

Nutritional Information:

➢ Total servings - 2 Per serving

➢ Fat: 42g

➢ Carbohydrates: 9g

➢ Protein: 29g

➢ Calories: 519

21) Keto baked apples

Ingredients:

- 2-ounce margarine
- 4 tbsp coconut flour
- 1-ounce walnuts
- ½ tbsp ground cinnamon
- One sharp apple
- ¾ cup substantial whipping cream
- 0.75 tbsp vanilla concentrate

Instructions:

1. Combine coconut, nuts, margarine, vanilla concentrate, and cinnamon to frame a batter.
2. Placed scaled-down bits of apple on a container lubed with oil.
3. Pour batter over the bits of apple.
4. Bake in a preheated stove at 350 degrees for 15 mins.
5. Mix half tbsp vanilla concentrate and whipping cream and beat until it gets soft.
6. Serve top heated apples with whipping cream and serve.

Nutritional Fact:

- Total Time: 20 mins
- Serving: 4
- Calories 340 kcal
- Proteins 3 g
- Carbohydrates 6 g

- ➢ Cholesterol 85 g
- ➢ Fat 33 g

22) Keto bagel recipe

Ingredients:

- ➢ 2 tbsp all that bagel preparing
- ➢ 1 cup cheddar
- ➢ 2eggs
- ➢ 1/2 cup parmesan cheddar ground

Instructions:

1. Whisk egg and cheddar in a bowl.
2. Pour in a doughnut container lubed with oil.
3. Drizzle flavoring over the egg blend.
4. Bake in a preheated stove at 375 degrees for 20 mins.

Nutritional Fact:

- ➢ Time: 17 mins
- ➢ Serving: 6
- ➢ Calories 218 kcal
- ➢ Proteins 14 g
- ➢ Carbohydrates 3 g
- ➢ Cholesterol 104 g
- ➢ Fat 16 g

23) Keto southwestern breakfast skillet

Ingredients:

- ➢ Four pieces of cut bacon
- ➢ 1/4 tbsp dark pepper

- ➢ 1/2 hacked onion
- ➢ 1/2 tbsp stew powder
- ➢ 1/2 tbsp spread
- ➢ One diced avocado
- ➢ 1/2 tbsp cumin
- ➢ 1/4 tbsp salt
- ➢ Four eggs
- ➢ 8 ounce cut radishes
- ➢ 1.25 cups hacked chime peppers
- ➢ 1/4 cup packed cilantro

Instructions:

1. In a huge, measured skillet, cook bacon.
2. Take out the bacon when it becomes firm and saved.
3. Chop the bacon when they get chill off.
4. In a similar container, over medium fire, cook onion and radish for five mins.
5. Add half tbsp of oil whenever required.
6. Add hacked ringer pepper and cook for the following four mins.
7. Add salt, stew powder, and dark pepper.
8. Make very nearly four spaces by siding the veggies and pour the egg in those spaces.
9. Cover the dish and cook for five mins. Mood killer the fire
10. Sprinkle hacked bacon, avocado, and cilantro and serve.

Nutritional Fact:

- ➢ Total Time: 35 mins

- ➢ Serving: 4
- ➢ Calories 253 kcal
- ➢ Proteins 12.5 g
- ➢ Carbohydrates 11 g
- ➢ Cholesterol 72 g
- ➢ Fat 18.5 g

24) Keto Banana Pancakes

Ingredients:

- ➢ 1 tbsp cinnamon
- ➢ Two bananas
- ➢ ½ tbsp preparing pop
- ➢ Four eggs

Instructions:

1. Combine all the fixings in a bowl.
2. In a dish, dissolve spread over medium warmth.
3. Place a spoonful blend in the container and cook for a little from the two sides while covering the dish.
4. Serve with coconut cream.

Nutritional Fact:

- ➢ Total Time: 15 mins
- ➢ Serving: 4
- ➢ Calories 117 kcal
- ➢ Proteins 6 g
- ➢ Carbohydrates 14 g
- ➢ Cholesterol 164 g

> Fat 4 g

25) Keto BLT lettuce wraps

Ingredients:

> Two cuts of lettuce

> Four cut tomato

> Four cuts cooked of bacon

> Black pepper to taste

> 1 tbsp mayonnaise

> salt to taste

Instructions:

1. Take each lettuce in turn and spot it over a plain surface.

2. Spread mayonnaise over lettuce leaves, place two bacon cuts, and tomato.

3. Drizzle pepper and salt over tomatoes and wrap the leave and serve.

Nutritional Fact:

> Total Time: 15 mins

> Serving: 2

> Calories 336 kcal

> Proteins 8 g

> Carbohydrates 2.7 g

> Cholesterol 42.8 g

> Fat 32.7 g

26) Cream cheese scrambled eggs

Ingredients:

> 2 tbsp spread

- ➢ Two eggs
- ➢ 1 tbsp whipping cream
- ➢ One squeeze pepper
- ➢ 2 tbsp cream cheddar
- ➢ One squeeze salt

Instructions:

1. Whisk cream, pepper, eggs, and salt in a bowl.
2. Melt spread in a container and pour egg blend in it.
3. Mix cream cheddar.
4. When the egg blend begins to set from the edges, overlay it to permit the fluid under the stream.
5. Cook until the blend is set as wanted and serve.

Nutritional Fact:

- ➢ Calories 181 kcal
- ➢ Proteins 8 g
- ➢ Carbohydrates 1.3 g
- ➢ Cholesterol 0 g
- ➢ Fat 16 g

27) Keto coconut porridge

Ingredients:

- ➢ One squeeze of psyllium husk powder
- ➢ 4 tbsp coconut cream
- ➢ 1 egg
- ➢ 1 squeeze salt
- ➢ 1 tbsp coconut flour
- ➢ 1oz spread

Instructions:

1. Whisk coconut flour, salt, egg, and husk powder.

2. In a dish, liquefy coconut cream and margarine.

3. Slowly pour egg blend with consistent mixing to get a thick combination.

4. Take out in a serving dish.

5. With coconut milk, serve the porridge.

Nutritional Fact:

➢ Total Time: 10 mins

➢ Serving: 1

➢ Calories 481 kcal

➢ Proteins 9 g

➢ Carbohydrates 4 g

➢ Cholesterol 30 g

➢ Fat 48 g

28) Keto Sausage with Creamy Basil Sauce

Ingredients:

➢ 8-ounce mozzarella

➢ 3 lb. Italian chicken wiener

➢ ¼ cup basil pesto

➢ 8-ounce cream cheddar

➢ ¼ cup hefty cream

Instructions:

1. Place wiener in a lubed dish and prepare for 30 mins in a preheated broiler at 400 degrees.

2. Mix well hefty cream, pesto, and cream cheddar.

3. Pour the rich sauce over the prepared hotdog.

4. Spread mozzarella cheddar over the top and prepare for an additional ten mins.

Nutritional Fact:

➢ Total Time: 45 mins

➢ Serving: 8

➢ Calories 436 kcal

➢ Proteins 28 g

➢ Carbohydrates 2 g

➢ Cholesterol 146g

➢ Fat 46 g

29) Cheesy Keto garlic bread

Ingredients:

➢ Bread with garlic

➢ 1/2 tsp of salt

➢ 3 eggs

➢ 3 tbsps powder of psyllium husk

➢ 1 tsp powder for baking

➢ 1 tsp of onion powder

➢ 1 cup of mozzarella cheese grated

➢ 1/2 cup of flour of coconut

➢ 1 tsp powder of garlic

➢ 1 cup of hot water

➢ 1 tsp of oregano

➢ 1 cup of flour of almond

Butter on Garlic

- ➢ 1/2 chopped cloves of garlic
- ➢ 1/4 cup of butter
- ➢ 1/2 tbsp of oregano
- ➢ 1/2 tsp of salt
- ➢ tbsps Parmesan shredded cheese

Instructions:

1. Combine half a tbsp of minced garlic, half a tbsp of oregano, half a tbsp of salt, half a cup of butter, and two tbsps of cheese.

2. Mix all the garlic bread ingredients, except water and egg, in a mixing bowl.

3. Mix the flour with the eggs and mix well to make the crumbled dough.

4. Then add water and blend to get a smooth, firm dough.

5. Set it in a baking dish and roll the dough into a sheet.

6. Bake at 350 degrees for 20 mins in a preheated oven.

7. Brush the top of the bread after baking with a garlic butter mixture and sprinkle the mozzarella cheese over the bread.

8. Bake once again and serve for 20 mins.

Nutritional Fact:

- ➢ Total Time: 60 mins
- ➢ Serving: 10 slices
- ➢ Calories 197 kcal
- ➢ Proteins 9 g
- ➢ Carbohydrates 8.5 g
- ➢ Cholesterol 72 g
- ➢ Fat 15 g

30) Keto seeded bread

Ingredients:

- ➤ 3 tbsps of sesame seeds
- ➤ 2 cups of almond flour
- ➤ 2 tbsps olive oil
- ➤ 1/4 tsp of salt
- ➤ 7 eggs
- ➤ 2 tbsps of chia seeds
- ➤ 1/2 tsp of xanthan gum
- ➤ 1/2 cup of butter
- ➤ 1 tsp powder for baking

Instructions:

1. Whisk the eggs together in a cup.

2. Chia seeds, baking powder, xanthan gum, sugar, salt, oil, and almond flour are whisked into the egg mixture using an electric beater.

3. Pour the batter and drizzle the sesame seeds into the baking pan.

4. Bake at 355 degrees for 40 mins in a preheated oven.

5. Slice the bread after cooling and store it in the fridge.

Nutritional Fact:

- ➤ Total Time: 50 mins
- ➤ Serving: 16
- ➤ Calories 175 kcal
- ➤ Proteins 6 g
- ➤ Carbohydrates 4 g

- ➤ Cholesterol 106 g
- ➤ Fat 16 g

31) Paleo and keto butter chicken

Ingredients:

- ➤ Marinade
- ➤ 1 tsp cumin powder
- ➤ 1 tbsp lemon juice
- ➤ Chicken 900 gs
- ➤ 2 tsp of turmeric powdered
- ➤ 1 cup of yogurt
- ➤ Salt to taste
- ➤ 1 tbsp of garam masala
- ➤ Butter Sauce
- ➤ One chopped jalapeno pepper
- ➤ 2 tbsps of almond flour
- ➤ One Onion Chopped
- ➤ 60 gs of butter
- ➤ 1 tbsp of grated ginger
- ➤ 1 cup of heavy cream
- ➤ 1/4 tsp cinnamon powder
- ➤ 1tbsp vegetable oil
- ➤ 14 oz of sliced tomatoes
- ➤ 1/2 cup of chicken broth
- ➤ Three chopped cloves of garlic
- ➤ Salt to taste

Instructions:

1. Combine the garam masala, salt, lemon juice, cumin, pepper, yogurt, and turmeric in a mixing bowl.

2. In a tub, add the chicken pieces and mix well so that the chicken is well coated.

3. For better results, put the bowl in the refrigerator overnight.

4. Heat the oil in a pan and add the butter.

5. Stir in the onions when the butter is melted and cook for 4 mins.

6. Mix the onion with the cinnamon, ginger, garlic, and cumin seeds and cook for an additional four mins.

7. Mix the salt, tomatoes, and chilies and cook for ten mins when the onions turn orange.

8. Mix the onion mixture with the chicken, including the marinade.

9. Add the broth after five mins of cooking, then bring it to a boil.

10. The pan is sealed and simmered for the next 15 mins.

11. Mix the almond flour and cream and simmer for another 15 mins.

12. By using salt and pepper, change the flavor accordingly.

13. For garnishing, use cilantro leaves.

Nutritional Fact:

➤ Total time: 60 mins

➤ Serving: 6

➤ Calories 367 kcal

➤ Proteins 36 gs

- ➢ Carbohydrates 7 gs
- ➢ Cholesterol 146 g
- ➢ Fat 22 gs

32) Baked Artichoke Hearts Au Gratin

Ingredients:

- ➢ 1/4 cup of almond flour
- ➢ 1/2 tsps puree of garlic
- ➢ 12 oz hearts of artichoke
- ➢ 1 Tbsp of lemon zest
- ➢ 1/4 cup of green onions chopped
- ➢ 1/4 Tsp dried oregano
- ➢ 2 Tbsps of olive oil
- ➢ 1/3 cup Pecorino-Romano shredded cheese
- ➢ Salting to taste
- ➢ 1/3 cup of Parmesan cheese grated
- ➢ 2 tbsps lemon juice
- ➢ 1/2 tsp dried thyme
- ➢ Black pepper to taste
- ➢ 1/3 cup of mayonnaise

Instructions:

1. Next, make the same-size slices of artichoke hearts.

2. Using oil to grease the baking tray.

3. Using a baking tray to create a single layer of artichoke hearts.

4. Drizzle over the top of the artichoke hearts with chopped onions, black pepper and salt.

5. Combine the shredded parmesan cheese, dried herbs, almond flour and pecorino romano cheese in a mixing bowl to create a fine, smooth paste.

6. Mix the lemon juice with the garlic puree, zest and mayonnaise.

7. Take half a cup of the mixture of cheese and blend in the garlic puree mixture.

8. Brush the mixture with the cheese over the artichoke hearts.

9. Cover with foil on the baking sheet.

10. Bake at 325 degrees for 30 mins in a preheated oven.

11. Spread the remaining cheese mixture over the artichoke hearts after 30 mins and bake at 375 degrees for another 25 mins.

12. Dish the artichoke hearts out and serve the dish while they are sweet.

Nutritional Fact:

- ➢ Total Time: 70 mins
- ➢ Serving: 4
- ➢ Calories 295 kcal;
- ➢ Proteins 9 g
- ➢ Carbohydrates 15 g
- ➢ Cholesterol 22 g
- ➢ Fat 24 g

33) Chicken green curry

Ingredients:

- ➢ 150 g of beansprouts
- ➢ Two chopped stalks of lemongrass

- ➢ 1 tbsp groundnut oil
- ➢ 1 tsp Thai sauce for fish
- ➢ Two Zest of Lemons
- ➢ 1/2 cup of chicken broth
- ➢ 700 g breast of chicken
- ➢ One diced clove of garlic
- ➢ Coriander as required for garnishing
- ➢ 200 g of green beans
- ➢ 1 tbsp lemon juice
- ➢ 13 oz of coconut milk
- ➢ Thai green curry paste 2 tbsp

Instructions:

1. In a pan, fry bite-sized chicken bits.

2. Add the curry paste, garlic, lemongrass, and lime zest when the chicken pieces have turned orange.

3. Cook and add chicken stock, coconut milk, and lime juice for 3 mins.

4. Cover it and let it simmer on a low flame for 10 mins.

5. Mix the green peas after 10 mins of simmering, then cook.

6. Combine the bean sprouts after two mins.

7. Switch off the flame after cooking for one min.

8. Garnish with coriander and serve with cauliflower rice.

Nutritional Fact:

- ➢ Total Time: 20 mins
- ➢ Serving: 4
- ➢ Calories 452 kcal

- ➢ Proteins 61 g
- ➢ Carbohydrates 7.5 g
- ➢ Cholesterol 158 g
- ➢ Fat 17 g

34) Keto beef kabobs

Ingredients:

Marinade

- ➢ 1 tsp powder of garlic
- ➢ 1 tsp of black pepper
- ➢ 2 tbsps olive oil
- ➢ 1 tsp of salt
- ➢ 1 tbsp of oregano
- ➢ 3 tbsps of vinegar (red wine)
- ➢ 1 tsp of onion powder
- ➢ 1 tsp of sauce Worcestershire

Cooking Steak

- ➢ 85 g of red, green, and yellow bell pepper for each
- ➢ Cube-shaped 1.5 lb. sirloin steaks
- ➢ 113 g red onion sliced
- ➢ 8 mushrooms

Instructions:

1. Combine the pepper, salt, oregano, garlic powder, Worcestershire sauce, vinegar, powdered onion and olive oil in a mixing bowl.

2. To get better results, add steak pieces and put them overnight in the fridge.

3. Thread beef alongside vegetables on a stick.

4. On medium heat, put a grill and heat the oil inside.

5. Over the grill, place threaded kabobs.

6. Brush the marinade over the kabobs regularly and continue changing the sides until both sides are fried.

Nutritional Fact:

- ➢ Total Time: 50 mins
- ➢ Serving: 8 kabobs
- ➢ Calories 168 kcal
- ➢ Proteins 19 g
- ➢ Carbohydrates 4 g
- ➢ Cholesterol 51 g
- ➢ Fat 7 g

35) Super simple braised red cabbage

Ingredients:

- ➢ 1/2 tsp ghee
- ➢ 2 tsp of erythritol (optional)
- ➢ 1/4 cup vinegar for cider (apple)
- ➢ One red onion sliced
- ➢ Black pepper to taste
- ➢ 2 tbsps of water
- ➢ Salt to taste
- ➢ 1/1 lb. of red cabbage chopped

Instructions:

1. Heat the ghee over a medium flame in a pan.

2. Sauté the onion for three mins in a pan.

3. Incorporate salt, erythritol, vinegar, chopped cabbage, pepper, and simmer for 7 mins.

4. Cover the pan after seven mins and cook on a low flame for 60 mins.

5. It can be kept in an air-tight container for up to five days.

Nutritional Fact:

- ➢ Total Time: 75 mins
- ➢ Serving: 4
- ➢ Calories 117 kcal
- ➢ Proteins 2 g
- ➢ Carbohydrates 7.9 g
- ➢ Cholesterol 10 g
- ➢ Fat 7.8 g

36) Labneh cheese ball

Ingredients:

- ➢ Flavored Oil
- ➢ 6 garlic cloves chopped
- ➢ 1/2 cup of olive oil
- ➢ 2 red chilies (dried)

For Labneh

- ➢ 3 tbsps of dill and mint chopped
- ➢ 1 tsp of salt
- ➢ 4- glasses of Greek yogurt

Instructions:

Flavoured Oil

1. Mix the chilies and garlic in a jar in a medium-sized mason jar.

2. To the pot, apply the olive oil and hold it for three days.

Labneh

1. To drain, pour yogurt into a strainer. Let it drain by leaving it in the refrigerator for three days.

2. Connect salt to the drained yogurt after three days and make small balls out of it.

3. Mix the finely chopped dill and mint in a dish.

4. Roll the yogurt balls to coat the balls in the dill and mint mixture.

5. Drop balls with flavored oil in a mason jar. When needed, add more olive oil.

6. Balls have to be completely dipped in grease.

7. Serve yogurt balls with vegetables or pita chips or bread on a serving plate.

Nutritional Fact:

- ➤ Total Time: 14 mins
- ➤ Serving: 6
- ➤ Calories 250 kcal
- ➤ Proteins 14 g
- ➤ Carbohydrates 7 g
- ➤ Cholesterol 0 g
- ➤ Fat 18 g

37) Keto Caesar salad

Ingredients:

- ➤ 2 tbsp of chopped anchovy
- ➤ 1 tbsp of mustard (Dijon)

- ➤ 1/4 cheese of parmesan (grated)
- ➤ Salt to taste
- ➤ Black pepper to taste
- ➤ One diced clove of garlic
- ➤ 1/2 cup of mayonnaise
- ➤ 1/2 lemon juice and zest
- ➤ Salad
- ➤ 7 oz of chopped lettuce
- ➤ 12 oz. breast of chicken
- ➤ 3 oz of bacon
- ➤ 1/2 cup of parmesan cheese (grated)
- ➤ 1 tbsp of olive oil
- ➤ Salt to taste
- ➤ Black pepper to taste

Instructions:

1. Mix the mustard, salt, lemon juice, cheese, anchovies, black pepper, garlic, lemon zest, and mayonnaise in an immersion mixer. Store it aside.

2. Place the chicken pieces and sprinkle them with black pepper, oil, and salt in a baking pan, greased with oil.

3. Bake the chicken for 20 mins at 350 degrees in a preheated oven.

4. Take a pan and fry the bacon in it while the chicken is in the oven.

5. Place some lettuce in a serving bowl.

6. Place the bacon and baked chicken pieces over the lettuce leaves and pour the pieces over the prepared dressing.

7. Garnish with and serve the grated cheese.

Nutritional Fact:

- ➢ Total Time: 35 mins
- ➢ Serving: 3
- ➢ Calories 997 kcal
- ➢ Proteins 71 g
- ➢ Carbohydrates 5 g
- ➢ Cholesterol 0g
- ➢ Fat 77 g

38) Chicken, spinach, and bacon salad

Ingredients:

- ➢ 1 cup of keto dressing ranch
- ➢ 150 g of spinach
- ➢ 1 cup of mushrooms chopped
- ➢ 5 Slices of Bacon
- ➢ 2 Breast Chicken
- ➢ 1 diced clove of garlic
- ➢ Basil as needed
- ➢ 4 tomatoes sun-dried
- ➢ 2 tsps olive oil

Instructions:

1. Heat the oil in a pan.
2. Garlic for cooking chicken until the chicken turns orange.
3. On a pan, take out the chicken bits.
4. Cook the bacon in the same pan.

5. In a dish, mix the bacon, chicken, mushrooms, spinach, and basil.

6. Spread the spinach into a serving dish and place the mixture of chicken and bacon over the spinach.

7. Drizzle the mixture with sun-dried tomatoes.

8. Store in the refrigerator for two days and use ranch dressing to serve.

Nutritional Fact:

➤ Total Time: 20 mins

➤ Serving: 3

➤ Calories 553 kcal

➤ Proteins 35 g

➤ Carbohydrates 3.3 g

➤ Cholesterol 0 g

➤ Fat 3.7 g

39) Keto broccoli salad

Ingredients:

➤ 2 tbsps of vinegar (apple cider)

➤ 1/2 cup of pumpkin seeds

➤ 8 sliced broccoli cups

➤ 1/2 lb. of bacon cooked and shredded

➤ 3/4 cup of mayonnaise

➤ 1/4 cup of red onion chopped

➤ Salt to taste

➤ 4 ounces of cheddar cheese

➤ Black pepper to taste

- ➢ 5 tsps of erythritol

Instructions:

1. Combine erythritol in a bowl with vinegar and mayonnaise. To get a smooth dressing combination, blend well.

2. Combine the pumpkin seeds, broccoli, cheese, and onion in a mixing bowl.

3. Pour the dressing into a bowl of broccoli mix.

4. Place the bowl in the refrigerator to cool and let the dressing and salad settle for three hours.

5. After drizzling with black pepper and salt, serve.

Nutritional Fact:

- ➢ Total Time: 10 mins
- ➢ Serving: 10
- ➢ Calories 266 kcal
- ➢ Proteins 8 g
- ➢ Carbohydrates 4 g
- ➢ Cholesterol 0 g
- ➢ Fat 25 g

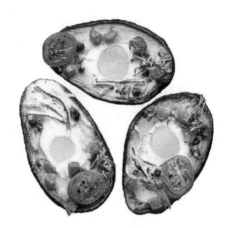

40) Keto Fried Eggs with Kale and Pork

Ingredients:

- ½ lbs kale
- 1 ounces cranberries
- 6-ounce pork belly smoked
- 1-ounce walnuts
- Salt to taste
- 3-ounce butter
- Four large eggs
- Pepper to taste

Instructions:

1. First sliced kale after trimming.
2. In a pan, melt butter (0.75 ounces) and add kale.

3. Cook on medium flame.

4. When kale edges turned brown, take out kale on a plate and set aside.

5. Add and cook pork in the same pan.

6. When pork becomes crispy, reduce the flame to low and add cooked kale walnuts and cranberries.

7. After the pan's content gets warm, then empty the pan in a serving bowl.

8. In the same pan, crack eggs separately in the remaining butter. Sprinkle black pepper and salt and fry to the desired level.

9. Put cooked eggs in a bowl with cooked pork, nuts, and kale and serve.

Nutritional Fact:

➢ Total Time: 20 mins

➢ Serving: 2

➢ Calories 1033 kcal

➢ Proteins 26 g

➢ Carbohydrates 8 g

➢ Cholesterol 141 g

➢ Fat 99 g

41) Halloumi Cheese Fingers

Ingredients:

➢ ½ tbsp olive oil

➢ tsps lemon juice

➢ 6 ounces halloumi cheese

➢ Pepper to taste

- ➤ ¼ tsps oregano

Instructions:

1. With a medium flame, heat olive oil in a saucepan.

2. Cook halloumi cheese for 2 mins or until turned brown.

3.Drizzle oregano, lemon juice, and black pepper and serve.

Nutritional Fact:

- ➤ Total Time: 10 mins
- ➤ Serving: 2
- ➤ Calories 299 kcal
- ➤ Proteins 18 gs
- ➤ Carbohydrates 3 gs
- ➤ Cholesterol 64 milligs
- ➤ Fat 25 gs

42) Mexican frittata

Ingredients:

- ➤ 1 tsp olive oil
- ➤ ¼ cup milk
- ➤ One sliced bell pepper (red)
- ➤ ½ salsa
- ➤ Two whole eggs
- ➤ One chopped white onion
- ➤ Four egg whites
- ➤ ½ tsp salt
- ➤ 1 tsp black pepper
- ➤ Pinch of cumin

Instructions:

1. , heat olive oil on medium in a skillet flame, sauté onion, and red bell pepper for about five mins.

2. In a mixing bowl, whisk eggs, egg white, milk, salt, cumin, and black pepper.

3. In a baking dish, place a stir-fried onion mixture.

4. Add egg mixture over onion and bell pepper mixture.

5. in a preheated oven at 350 degrees for 30 mins.

6. Make slices of the frittata and serve with salsa.

Nutritional Fact:

- ➢ Total Time: 50 mins
- ➢ Serving: 2
- ➢ Calories 202 kcal
- ➢ Proteins 17 g
- ➢ Carbohydrates 16 g
- ➢ Cholesterol 188 g
- ➢ Fat 8.5 g

43) Italian style baked eggs

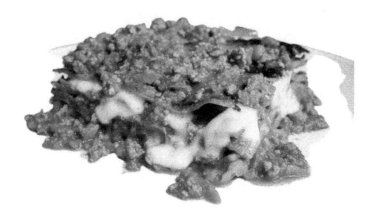

Ingredients:

- ➢ 4 ounces pancetta diced
- ➢ 5 eggs
- ➢ 1/4 tsp salt to taste
- ➢ 1/2 cup chopped onion
- ➢ 1/2 tsp chopped garlic
- ➢ 1/2 cup chopped tomato
- ➢ 1/4 cup almond milk
- ➢ 1/2 cup chopped oregano
- ➢ 1/2 cup chopped basil
- ➢ 1 cup tomato sauce

- ➢ Black pepper to taste
- ➢ Red pepper flakes for garnishing
- ➢ 2/3 cup grated parmesan cheese
- ➢ Oregano for garnishing

Instructions:

1. In a pan, add onion and pancetta in a skillet and sauté for two mins.

2. Turn off the flame

3. In a mixing bowl, add cheese and milk and whisk them well.

4. Add tomato, herbs, garlic, tomato sauce, black pepper, salt, and mix.

5. Add tomato mixture in skillet with pancetta and onion.

6. Placing eggs in the pan makes a small space using a spatula by moving the mixture aside.

7. Break eggs and pour them in spaces created in a mixture: one egg in each space.

8. Put some cheese on the upper surface.

9. For 15 mins ake in a preheated oven at 425 degrees

10. Use flakes and parsley to garnish and serve.

Nutritional Fact:

- ➢ Total Time: 28 mins
- ➢ Serving: 4
- ➢ Calories 207 kcal
- ➢ Proteins 14 g
- ➢ Carbohydrates 6 g
- ➢ Cholesterol 204 g
- ➢ Fat 14.4 gs

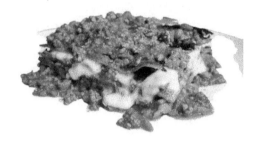

44) Halloumi Cheese Fingers

Ingredients:

- ½ tbsp olive oil
- 2 tsps lemon juice
- 6-ounce halloumi cheese
- Pepper to taste
- ¼ tsp oregano

Instructions:

1. With the gas on a medium flame, heat olive oil in a saucepan.

2. Cook halloumi cheese for 2 mins or until turned brown.

3. Drizzle oregano, lemon juice, and black pepper and serve.

Nutritional Fact:

- Total Time: 10 mins
- Serving: 2
- Calories 299 kcal
- Proteins 18 g
- Carbohydrates 3 g

- ➢ Cholesterol 64 g
- ➢ Fat 25 g

45) Mexican frittata

Ingredients:

- ➢ 1 tsp olive oil
- ➢ ¼ cup milk
- ➢ One sliced bell pepper (red)
- ➢ ½ salsa
- ➢ Two whole eggs
- ➢ One chopped white onion
- ➢ Four egg whites
- ➢ ½ tsp salt
- ➢ 1 tsp black pepper
- ➢ Pinch of cumin

Instructions:

1. heat olive oil on medium flame in a skillet, sauté onion, and red bell pepper for about five mins.

2. In a mixing bowl, whisk eggs, egg white, milk, salt, cumin, and black pepper.

3. In a baking dish, place a stir-fried onion mixture.

4. Add egg mixture over onion and bell pepper mixture.

5. place baking dish in a preheated oven at 350 degrees for 30 mins.

6. Make slices of the frittata and serve with salsa.

Nutritional Fact:

- ➢ Total Time: 50 mins

- Serving: 2
- Calories 202 kcal
- Proteins 17 g
- Carbohydrates 16 g
- Cholesterol 188 g
- Fat 8.5 g

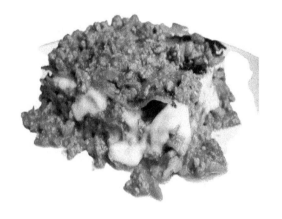

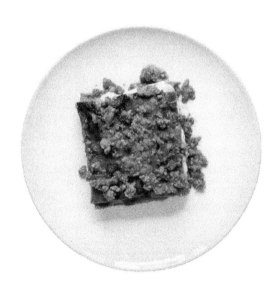

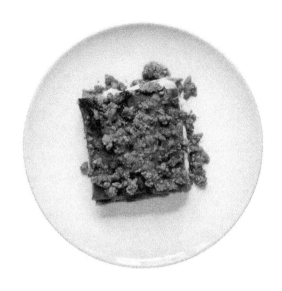

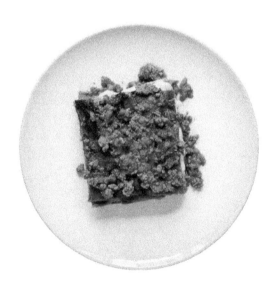

46) Italian style baked eggs

Ingredients:

- ➤ 4 ounces pancetta diced
- ➤ Five eggs
- ➤ 1/4 tsp salt to taste
- ➤ 1/2 cup chopped onion
- ➤ 1/2 tsp chopped garlic
- ➤ 1/2 cup chopped tomato
- ➤ 1/4 cup almond milk
- ➤ 1/2 cup chopped oregano
- ➤ 1/2 cup chopped basil
- ➤ 1 cup tomato sauce
- ➤ Black pepper to taste
- ➤ Red pepper flakes for garnishing
- ➤ 2/3 cup grated parmesan cheese
- ➤ Oregano for garnishing

Instructions:

1. In a pan, add onion and pancetta in a skillet and sauté for two mins.

2. Turn off the flame

3. In a mixing bowl, add cheese and milk and whisk them well.

4. Add tomato, herbs, garlic, tomato sauce, black pepper, salt, and mix.

5. Add tomato mixture in skillet with pancetta and onion.

6. Placing eggs in the pan makes a small space using a spatula by moving the mixture aside.

7. Break eggs and pour them in spaces created in a mixture: one egg in each space.

8. Put some cheese on the upper surface.

9. for 15 mins, bake in a preheated oven at 425 degrees

10. Use flakes and parsley to garnish and serve.

Nutritional Fact:

- ➢ Total Time: 28 mins
- ➢ Serving: 4
- ➢ Calories 207 kcal
- ➢ Proteins 14 g
- ➢ Carbohydrates 6 g
- ➢ Cholesterol 204 g
- ➢ Fat 14.4 g

47) Keto Stuffed Portobello Mushrooms

Ingredients:

- ➢ Four Portobello mushroom
- ➢ 1-ounce basil
- ➢ 4 ounces. cream cheese
- ➢ 1 tbsp Italian herb mixture
- ➢ Eight slices of provolone cheese
- ➢ 1 tsp salt
- ➢ 1 tsp minced garlic
- ➢ 1 tsp smoked paprika
- ➢ 24 ounces sliced black olives
- ➢ 1/2 tsp black pepper
- ➢ 1 tsp chopped onion

Instructions:

1. Whisk seasonings and cream cheese in a mixing bowl.

2. Pour cream cheese blend in a pan or small cups.

3. Place the second layer of one ounce of olives (sliced) on cream cheese mixture in cups.

4. Place the third layer of cheese.

5. Drizzle pepper or salt to enhance the flavor.

6. Cover the cups with foil.

7. Bake in a preheated oven at 425 degrees for 25 mins.

8. Garnish with basil leaves before serving.

Nutritional Fact:

- Total Time: 30 mins
- Serving: 4
- Calories 647 kcal
- Proteins 20 g
- Carbohydrates 5 g
- Cholesterol 30 g
- Fat 62 g

48) Keto broccoli cauliflower salad

Ingredients:

Amish salad

- ½ cup chopped onion
- 4 cup chopped broccoli and cauliflower stems and florets
- ¼ cup walnut
- Nine slices of chopped bacon

Amish dressing

- ½ tsp black pepper
- 1 cup mayonnaise
- tbsps sugar substitute
- ½ cup chopped onion
- 1 tsp salt
- 1 cup sour cream
- tbsp vinegar (apple cider)

Instructions:

1. Mix sweetener sour cream, onions, salt, mayonnaise, and pepper in a mixing bowl. The dressing is ready. Keep it aside.

2. In another bowl, mix broccoli and cauliflower and mix well.

3. Add dressing over the cauliflower mixture and toss to coat the vegetables with the dressing fully.

4. Add nuts and bacon and mix well.

5. It can store for three days in the refrigerator.

Nutritional Fact:

- Total Time: 25 mins
- Serving: 12
- Calories 118 kcal
- Proteins 4.2 g
- Carbohydrates 4.9 g
- Cholesterol 20 g
- Fat 9.1 g

49) Keto hamburger salad

Ingredients:

Sauce

- 1 tbsp chopped onions
- 3/4 cup Mayonnaise
- 1 tbsp vinegar
- 1/2 tsp paprika (smoked)
- 2tbsp Dill Pickles
- tsps swerve
- tsp Mustard

Salad

- 1 lb ground beef
- 1 cup cheddar cheese shredded
- 1 tsp kosher salt
- 4 cups lettuce chopped
- ½ cup onions sliced
- 1 tsp black pepper
- 1/4 cup dill pickles

Instructions:

1.   First, prepare the dressing by combining mustard, paprika, mayonnaise, onion, pickles, swerve, and vinegar in a bowl. Set aside.

2.   On medium flame, heat the pan, stir in ground beef and cook for 10 mins.

3.   Sprinkle pepper and salt and cook until beef is done.

4.   Mix onion, lettuce, cheese, and pickles in a bowl.

5.   Add beef to the mixture and pour dressing over the beef. Toss well to mix everything thoroughly.

6.   Serve.

Nutritional Fact:

- ➤ Total Time: 25 mins
- ➤ Serving: 4
- ➤ Calories 625 kcal
- ➤ Proteins 31 g
- ➤ Carbohydrates 5 g
- ➤ Cholesterol 0 g
- ➤ Fat 52 g

Conclusion

Accepting that the limitations of another eating routine can prove challenging at times, When it comes to food and plans often, they turn out to be so close to home and our families that it seems difficult to split away from them. Fortunately, there are simple approaches to make options in contrast to your number one food sources, so they fit inside keto, or if nothing else- stay inside a nearby window.

Assuming you do not experience any symptoms that come with medical conditions, a ketogenic diet can provide you with numerous advantages, particularly revolving around weight reduction. The main thing to retain is to eat an incredible equilibrium of vegetables, lean meat, and natural carbs.

In effect, adhering to the required nourishments is suggested to be the most proficient method for eating strongly, principally due to its simplicity and being a maintainable strategy. It is imperative to note that a great deal of exploration demonstrates that ketogenic slims down are hard to keep up with; Thus, the best yet effective solution is to locate a comfortable eating method that is suited to you. There are no stigmas around attempting new things, however, do not rush into it- take your time.

Ketones are at the focal point of the ketogenic diet- Your body produces ketones, a fuel particle, as an elective fuel source when the body lacks glucose. The process of delivering ketones happens when you decrease carbs and devour the perfect measure of protein.

When you have reached the point where you are eating keto compliant food products, your liver can convert muscle to fat ratio into ketones, where following this, it gets utilized as a fuel source by your body. At the point where the body is utilizing fat as a fuel source, you have entered ketosis. It permits the body to increase its rate of fat consumption significantly now and again. Furthermore, this helps with lessening pockets of undesirable fat.

This fat consumption technique not exclusively helps you shed lbs, but it can likewise avoid yearnings and forestall energy crashes for the day.

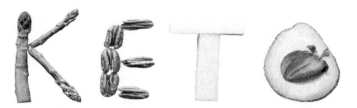